GW00854291

The Li

David M Hinds

Published by Community Health Publishing CHP
Crumplehorn Mill, Polperro, Cornwall PL13 2RJ
Telephone: 01503 273074   Fax: 01503 273148
e-mail: david@chpublishing.fslife.co.uk

First published in Great Britain in 2003

Published by Community Health Publishing CHP
Crumplehorn Mill, Polperro, Cornwall PL13 2RJ
Telephone: 01503 273074   Fax: 01503 273148
e-mail: david@chpublishing.fslife.co.uk

CHP is a non profit-making organisation created to assist seriously
ill patients make the best possible recovery available to them

ISBN: 0-9544285-0-1

Printed and bound in Great Britain by intype LONDON LTD,
Units 3/4, Elm Grove Industrial Estate, Wimbledon SW19 4HE

Other health titles by David M Hinds

After Stroke, published by Thorsons in the UK @ £9.99 and HarperCollins in the USA @ $15.99, is the UK's *top-selling title on stroke. This warm and motivating book is easy to read and opens with a foreword by Professor Sir Peter J Morris.

Beat Depression, published by Hodder and Stoughton @ £6.99, is uplifting and inspirational, enabling readers to help themselves at a time when they may be lethargic or experiencing uncomfortable emotions.

*Source: Amazon 2000/2001/2002

Acknowledgements

I would like to thank 7 people in particular for their enthusiasm and support during the writing of this book and for their appraisal of the early drafts of the manuscript.

Many thanks to Dot Rowles at the Women's Royal Voluntary Service, Liz Louch at the National Association of Hospital and Community Friends, Tony Kyriakides-Yeldham at Plymouth Hospitals NHS Trust, Derek Campbell, my mentor in this undertaking, Andrew and Jo-Anne Taylor at the Crumplehorn Mill, and to my wife, Tatiana.

I am also indebted to Jayne Hathway and the Scarman Trust SW and to Andréa Leplae and the Community Champions Fund South West for their assistance in bringing this project to fruition.

Introduction

When you are seriously ill or injured the last thing you feel like is the effort of reading a conventional book. But this warmly personal and patient-friendly little book, by an author who has suffered two devastating strokes and recovered using techniques he employed as an award-winning stress counsellor, will inspire and motivate readers to make the best possible recovery available.

Please note that this book is not intended to be a substitute for medical advice or treatment. Any person with a medical condition should consult a qualified medical practitioner.

Relax. Don't worry

Illness is the night-side of life… Everyone who is born holds dual citizenship, in the kingdom of the well and in the kingdom of the sick. Although we all prefer to use only the good passport, sooner or later each of us is obliged, at least for a spell, to identify ourselves as citizens of that other place.

Susan Sontag, b.1933, Illness as Metaphor

Relax. Don't worry

Try not to worry unnecessarily about your condition. Relax and allow the recuperative process to begin or *accelerate*. In the pages to come you will discover valuable tips to help you deal positively with the night-side of life.

THE BOTTOM LINE

Be gentle with yourself

Power

Power is the ultimate aphrodisiac.

Henry Kissinger, b.1923, The New York Times

Power

Within us, we harbour recuperative powers that need stimulation to be awakened. The key to this power is within our thoughts. Imagine, as you lay motionless and receptive to new ideas in bed, that you have access to your own internal physician who is going to work painlessly with you overnight to lay the foundations for you to cure your ills.

THE BOTTOM LINE

Access the power within

Shared experience

The arts then act like a reflecting mirror. The artist is like the hand that holds and moves the mirror, this way and that way, to explore all corners of the universe. But what is reflected in the mirror depends on where the holder stands...

Ngugi wa Thiongo, b.1938, Barrel of a Pen

Shared experience

There are times when a patient needs to know that at least one other has encountered and come through a similar experience. How that message is conveyed - through the arts, in print, or in person - is not important because the only qualification that matters is shared experience.

THE BOTTOM LINE

I have been where you are now

Gaining in strength

The world breaks everyone and afterward
many are strong at the broken places.

Ernest Hemingway, 1898–1961, Farewell to Arms

Gaining in strength

It is my privilege to have worked with many people who, after confronting their worst fears, emerge from the crisis stronger and more secure. You, too, can gain strength from your ordeal by trusting in your ability to cope and by using this book for inspiration and support.

THE BOTTOM LINE

You can be strong

Managing your recovery

The world is disgracefully managed,
one hardly knows to whom to complain.

Ronald Firbank, 1886–1926, Mrs Shamefoot in
Vainglory

Managing your recovery

In hospital or during periods of convalescence it is easy to feel you have lost control of your day-to-day existence. Although you cannot be in of control of everything, don't allow yourself to feel like a victim. This is merely a passing phase in your life.

THE BOTTOM LINE

The next phase will be better

Self-healing strategy

A man's greatest battles are the ones he fights
within himself

Ben Okri, b.1959, Flowers and Shadows

Self-healing strategy

Last thing at night, when all is quiet, tell yourself that what you want is the best recovery available to you. Reinforce this desire and impress it upon your mind by saying it again and again with conviction and you will succeed in accessing powerful parts of your mind that you may never have used before.

THE BOTTOM LINE

Harness subconscious energy

A reason to get better

Nothing contributes so much to tranquillise the mind as a steady purpose: a point on which the soul may fix its intellectual eye.

Mary Shelley, 1797–1851, Frankenstein

A reason to get better

A patient with a passion for life and a mission to fulfil is a patient who is very likely to make the best recovery available. Focus your mind on a realisable dream and you mobilise the forces of mind and body in turning back disease.

THE BOTTOM LINE

You have a mission to fulfil

Strike gold from your sickbed

Whatever you can do, or dream you can, begin it.
Boldness has genius, power and magic in it.

Goethe, 1749 – 1832

Strike gold from your sickbed

For better or for worse, we all ultimately direct our own lives. After two major strokes and a subclavian bypass, I dreamed of writing a book - *After Stroke*. Within four years I had made a complete recovery, and in the fifth year the book was published on both sides of the Atlantic.

THE BOTTOM LINE

Benefit from your misfortune

Hope

Hope is a waking dream

Aristotle, circa 384–322 BC, Lives and Opinions of
Eminent Philosophers

Hope

Even when confronted with the inevitable setbacks along the uphill return to health, never give up on your dream of getting well. As long as you continue to nurture your desire for recovery with undying passion and belief, there is always the opportunity of fulfilment.

THE BOTTOM LINE

Hope for recovery

Therapeutic success

Christian Science is so often therapeutically successful because it lays stress on the patient's believing in his or her own health rather than in Noah's Ark…

J B S Haldane, 1892–1964, Possible Worlds,
"Duty of Doubt"

Therapeutic success

Accident and disease have their own special way of concentrating the mind on what really matters in life. Consider how best to cope with or cure your present disorder and do what you can to minimise any disadvantages or disabilities.

THE BOTTOM LINE

Success may come sooner than expected

The beauty of chaos

Chaos often breeds life, when order breeds habit.

Henry Adams, 1838–1918, The Education of Henry Adams

The beauty of chaos

Survivors of life-threatening illnesses who recovered their health by eliminating disease-generating habits and by reforming their lifestyle and diet, know that chaos brings change and change commences with one simple step: the first step.

THE BOTTOM LINE

Take the first step

Let go of anger

What other dungeon is so dark as one's own heart!
What jailer so inexorable as one's self!

Nathaniel Hawthorne, 1804–1864, The House of the
Seven Gables

Let go of anger

Let go of anger - it is a dangerous and corrosive acid that burns away at the delicate layers of your peace of mind. Forgiveness is the greatest healer.

THE BOTTOM LINE

Forgive yourself, as well as others

Think like a genius

Someone who has completely lost his way in a forest, but strives with uncommon energy to get out of it in whatever direction, sometimes discovers a new, unknown way: this is how geniuses come into being, who are then praised for their originality.

Friedrich Nietzsche, 1844–1900, Human, All Too Human

Think like a genius

Instead of allowing your mind to freeze up in the wake of accident or serious illness like a deer in the headlights, entertain the prospect of finding a new and original way to prosper from your predicament.

THE BOTTOM LINE

Be original

High adventure

The growth of the human mind is still high adventure, in many ways the highest adventure on earth.

Norman Cousins (who was diagnosed as *terminally ill* with odds against survival of 500/1, recovered in full... How? By demonstrating a remarkable will to live and by discovering, through trial and error, that laughter brought him relief from pain and developing this theme into laughter therapy), 1915–1990, Anatomy Of An Illness *As Perceived By The Patient*

High adventure

Why not suppose that the forthcoming struggle to recover your health will be an adventure, an opportunity to strengthen your character, as well as your body? We learn more about ourselves from the painful experiences in life than we do from the periods of ecstasy.

THE BOTTOM LINE

Embrace this adventure

Water

Water is best
(Inscription over the Pump Room, Bath)

Pindar, 518 – c. 437 BC, Olympian Odes

Water

Water - plain, ordinary tap water (as well as the bottled variety) - has tremendous healing power and can guard against allergies, depression, high blood pressure, and even certain types of cancer. Several glasses a day are ideal. Try it on a regular basis and see how much better you feel!

THE BOTTOM LINE

Water possesses healing qualities

The audition

The important thing in acting is to be able to laugh and cry. If I have to cry, I think of my sex life. If I have to laugh, I think of my sex life...

Glenda Jackson, b.1936

The audition

Imagine you were in Hollywood auditioning for the starring role in the forthcoming movie, *Against All Odds.* In order to get the part you are required to smile your warmest smile, then laugh in the face of adversity; what will inspire you to give an Oscar-winning performance?

THE BOTTOM LINE

The director is waiting...

Peace of mind

I expect to pass through this world but once; any good thing therefore that I can do, or any kindness that I can show to any fellow-creature, let me do it now; let me not defer or neglect it, for I shall not pass this way again.

{Attributed to} Stephen Grellet, 1773–1855

Peace of mind

Peace of mind is the great facilitator in recovery. Our mind and body communicate constantly with each other - mainly at an unconscious level - and a peaceful mind allows the body to heal more effectively.

THE BOTTOM LINE

Be kind to yourself, and others

Poetry

All poetry is a journey into the unknown.

Vladimir Mayakovsky, 1893–1930,
Poem: A Conversation with the Inspector of Taxes

Poetry

The surest way I know, for poets and non-poets alike, to extract the poison from fear and render it naked, impotent, and ridiculous, is to set about putting it to poetry. Something in the process of writing starts to draw out the venom.

THE BOTTOM LINE

Write your poem

Simplify your life

Most of the evils in life arise from man's being
unable to sit still in a room.

Blaise Pascal, 1623–1662, Pensées

Simplify your life

Avoid reducing your chances of total recovery by maintaining too many responsibilities and *"carrying on regardless"*. The only thing that matters right now is getting well and anything that conflicts with that one overriding priority should take a back seat for a while.

THE BOTTOM LINE

KISS (*K*eep *I*t *S*imple *S*exy)

Be positive

The life of nations no less than that of men is lived largely in the imagination.

Enoch Powell, 1912–1998

Be positive

A positive mental attitude and a lively imagination can influence the body's immune system, which in turn affects how well we fight disease. What you believe and what you are capable of imagining can have a far-reaching effect on your own body and its ability to go into remission or repair itself.

THE BOTTOM LINE

Dare to imagine the finest outcome

Problems

A moment's insight is sometimes worth a life's experience

Oliver Wendell Holmes senior, 1809–94,
The Professor at the Breakfast Table

Problems

There has never been, nor will there ever be, a life free from problems. It is not the presence, scale, or magnitude of problems but how we tackle them that determines the quality of our lives.

THE BOTTOM LINE

Problems are best handled *without* emotion

Internal clatter

My mind is troubled like a fountain stirred;
And I myself see not the bottom of it.

William Shakespeare, 1564–1616,
Troilus and Cressida

Internal clatter

When we are troubled by health matters, internal clatter - in the form of negative thoughts, doubts, and unhelpful murmurings - surface inside our heads. We can counter this by slowly repeating to ourselves, with as much certainty as possible, "I will be OK."

THE BOTTOM LINE

*"**I will be OK**."* Say it!

Let your worries melt like ice

Before the cherry orchard was sold everybody was worried and upset, but as soon as it was all settled... everybody calmed down, and felt quite cheerful.

Anton Chekhov, 1860–1904, The Cherry Orchard

Let your worries melt like ice

Ice melts without any input from mankind. Relaxed and enlightened people know that there has never been, nor will there be, a problem solved by worrying so they leave their worries to simply melt away like ice.

THE BOTTOM LINE

Worrying is a waste of time

Be patient. Give recovery a chance

Patience and passage of time do more than
strength and fury.

Jean de La Fontaine, 1621–1695, Le Lion et le Rat,
Fables bk. 2

Be patient. Give recovery a chance

We all have legitimate concerns but fretting about them will slow your recovery. A worried mind can interfere with the body's ability to combat disease and repair itself by adversely affecting the central nervous system, the endocrine system, and the immune system. Be patient and allow recovery to happen.

THE BOTTOM LINE

Patience is the elixir of life

Enjoyment

I am a woman who enjoys herself very much;
sometimes I lose, sometimes I win.

Mata Hari, 1876–1917, Mata Hari, The True Story

Enjoyment

The essential thing about life is to enjoy it; not only the high spots, but through ill-health and the inevitable setbacks along the way towards fulfilment and peace of mind.

THE BOTTOM LINE

Enjoy your journey through life

Reward

Great thoughts come from the heart... The most absurd and the most rash hopes have sometimes been the cause of extraordinary success.

Marquis de Vauvenargues, 1715–47,
Reflections and Maxims

Reward

When I was ill, I booked myself a holiday in Rio de Janeiro (to the horror and disbelief of my doctor *and* my travel agent) to commence several months after my operation. Rio was my reason to get well and my reward for getting well!

THE BOTTOM LINE

Choose your reward!

| You are not alone |

Although the world is full of suffering, it is full also of the overcoming of it.

Helen Keller, 1880–1968

You are not alone

When serious illness strikes, fear, self-doubt, and anxiety conspire to suck the energy and optimism out of some patients. Initially, they may feel helpless and unable to cope. Now that you have become acquainted with this little book, accept it as a friend to be browsed through at leisure and you will be surprised how well you manage.

THE BOTTOM LINE

Read on and feel your confidence rise

Change

In spite of illness, in spite even of the archenemy sorrow, one can remain alive long past the usual date of disintegration if one is unafraid of change.

Edith Wharton, 1862–937, A Backward Glance

Change

Change is best managed if you embrace it. To my astonishment and subsequent delight, my new life that was forced upon me by stroke is better and more rewarding.

THE BOTTOM LINE

Change may surprise and delight you!

Misunderstandings

We do not see things as they are.
We see things as we are.

The Talmud, circa AD 500

Misunderstandings

Whenever two people meet there are really six people present. There is each man as he sees himself, each man as the other person sees him and each man as he really is.

William James, 1842–1910

THE BOTTOM LINE

Make allowances for the others!

Sorrow

Telling one's sorrows often brings comfort.

Pierre Corneille, 1606–84, Polyeucte

Sorrow

Can I see another's woe, and not be in sorrow too.
Can I see another's grief, and not seek for kind relief.

William Blake, 1757 - 1827, Songs of Innocence

THE BOTTOM LINE

Talking can bring comfort and relief

The birth of spring

Weeping may endure for a night, but joy cometh
in the morning.

Psalms 30:5

The birth of spring

If your illness is making you unhappy, think of your unhappiness as a winter, the time of year we regard as bleak and infertile, but which is really the season that prepares us for life, and gives birth to spring.

THE BOTTOM LINE

You will feel better in time

Conversation

Conversation has a kind of charm about it, an insinuating and insidious something that elicits secrets from us just like love or liqueur.

Seneca, 4 BC–AD 65, Epistles

Conversation

Why not surprise a friend or relative by telephoning them? Or you could bring a smile to someone's face right now by complimenting him or her. If you are in a nursing home, or recovering in hospital, speak kindly to someone nearby.

THE BOTTOM LINE

It's good to talk

The tickle of mirth

'Tis a good thing to laugh at any rate; and if a straw can tickle a man, it is an instrument of happiness.

John Dryden, 1631–1700,
A Parallel of Poetry and Painting

The tickle of mirth

Mirth is like a flash of lightning, that breaks through a gloom of clouds, and glitters for a moment; cheerfulness keeps up a kind of daylight in the mind, and fills it with a steady and perpetual serenity.

Joseph Addison, 1672–1719, The Spectator No. 381 (17th May, 1712)

THE BOTTOM LINE

Laughter breaks through the gloom

Reflections

Our life is what our thoughts make it

Marcus Aurelius, AD 121–180, Meditations

Reflections

Take a few moments to reflect on what you have been doing, and what you will do in the future, to aid your recovery. Don't forget to give yourself a huge helping of well-deserved praise for taking the trouble to read this book.

THE BOTTOM LINE

Reflect and congratulate. You're doing OK

The honey couch

Words may be false and full of art;
sighs are the natural language of the heart.

Thomas Shadwell, 1642–92, Psyche

The honey couch

When life is tough and you find yourself in unfamiliar surroundings, retreat to the honey couch - a room, a chair, even a different position on your pillow will suffice - anywhere you can relax and sigh your heart out when you feel the need.

THE BOTTOM LINE

Relax on the honey couch

Feed your imagination

His imagination resembled the wings of an ostrich. It enabled him to run, though not to soar.

Lord Macaulay, 1800–1859,
commenting on John Dryden, 1631–1700 {in 1828}

Feed your imagination

Your imagination is more active and fertile when you are participating in something, as indeed you are doing now by reading this book. Conversely, it has a tendency to be stunted and dulled by being a passive spectator.

THE BOTTOM LINE

Life can be a dream come true

Wellbeing

Wellbeing is attained little and little, and nevertheless it is no little thing itself.

Zeno of Citium (4th–3rd century BC),
Lives and Opinions of Eminent Philosophers

Wellbeing

If there is something you have always yearned to do, but never attempted, plan to do it just as soon as you are well enough. This, more than anything else, will hasten your recovery and bring about a feeling of wellbeing.

THE BOTTOM LINE

Be yourself: the self you always wanted

Get high on a banana

The art of medicine consists of amusing the patient while nature cures the disease.

Voltaire, 1694–1778

Get high on a banana

Foods high in potassium, such as bananas and kiwi fruit, are reputed to encourage feelings of wellbeing and cheerfulness. How often have you seen a depressed monkey?

THE BOTTOM LINE

Peel it and *get high!*

Plonk

It was my uncle George who discovered that alcohol was a food well in advance of modern medical thought.

P G Wodehouse, 1881–1975, The Inimitable Jeeves

Plonk

A glass of red wine a day (any red wine - even plonk!) can be good for you because the grape skins used in the fermentation process produce blood-thinning agents that reduce the risk of heart disease, blood clots and stroke. Wine also kills bacteria and viruses, raises good HDL blood cholesterol, and is rich in chemicals that help to prevent cancer.

THE BOTTOM LINE

One glass of red wine each day? *Cheers!*

Accelerate your recovery

I know of no more encouraging fact than the unquestionable ability of man to elevate his life by conscious endeavour.

Henry David Thoreau, 1817–1862, Walden

Accelerate your recovery

Your mind is capable of making the best or the worst of any situation, depending on your attitude and frame of mind. Set your mind to making the best possible recovery available to you and prepare to surprise yourself.

THE BOTTOM LINE

Your best will do very well indeed

Smile

When you're smiling the whole world smiles with
you.

Joe Goodwin, 1889–1943 and Larry Shay, 1897–1988,
song: When You're Smiling

Smile

A smile exercises and tones your facial muscles by tensing then relaxing them. It makes you feel good emotionally and physically and it can be heart-warming for others to see.

THE BOTTOM LINE

One smile can make all the difference

Hard times

The greatness of human actions is measured by
the extent to which they inspire others.

Louis Pasteur, 1822–1895

Hard times

Some years back, when I was almost broken and defeated, someone I greatly admired, said, "David, one day you will look back at this chapter in your life and laugh". I thought he was heartless; in fact, he was right.

THE BOTTOM LINE

Your day to chuckle will come

Bitter thoughts

If we could read the secret history of our enemies, we should find in each man's life sorrow and suffering enough to disarm hostility.

Henry Wadsworth Longfellow, 1807–1882, Driftwood

Bitter thoughts

So many people, while coping adequately or even bravely with tragedy or ill-health, allow themselves to be brought down by bitter thoughts - *what he or she did or did not say or do!* Dispense with these trivialities which can hurt you only if you continue to remember them.

THE BOTTOM LINE

Forgive and forget

Loss of faith

The most wonderful thing about Saints is that they were human. They lost their tempers, got angry, scolded God... made mistakes and regretted them. Still they went on doggedly blundering towards heaven.

Phyllis McGinley, 1905–1978

Loss of faith

Occasionally, when religious people meet with the tragedy of serious illness, they cannot believe that God would allow this to happen to them and they are tempted to lose faith. If this theme is relevant to you, recognise that the quest for fulfilment cannot be without challenges and obstacles.

THE BOTTOM LINE

Could this setback be a test of faith?

"How long have I got, Doctor?"

Who shall decide when doctors disagree?

Alexander Pope, 1688–1744, Moral Essays

"How long have I got, Doctor?"

Predictions can prove to be correct or wildly inaccurate because the mental attitude of the individual is paramount. Naturally, some patients die as anticipated, others succeed in extending their lives, and some go on to make a complete and spontaneous recovery, contrary to expert expectation.

THE BOTTOM LINE

Predictions can be wrong

The placebo effect

Optimistic lies have such immense therapeutic value that a doctor who cannot tell them convincingly has mistaken his profession.

George Bernard Shaw, 1856–1950
Misalliance

The placebo effect

More than 1 in 4 patients in the UK who are prescribed placebos (drugs with no active ingredients - chalk powder, to you and me!) get better merely because *they believe* they are taking an effective remedy. This placebo effect is proof positive that in many cases your mind is capable of causing your body to heal itself when prompted into action by belief.

THE BOTTOM LINE

Believe in something!

Enjoying the moment

This is no cure for birth and death
save to enjoy the interval.

George Santayana, 1863–1952

Enjoying the moment

Happy the man, and happy he alone,
He, who can call today his own:
He who, secure within, can say,
Tomorrow do thy worst, for I have lived today.

John Dryden, 1631–1700
From a translation of Horace, circa 65–8 BC

THE BOTTOM LINE

Enjoy life as best you can

Creative convalescence

There are some days when I think I'm going to die
from an overdose of satisfaction.

Salvador Dali, 1904–1989

Creative convalescence

Time spent in creative activities such as art, chess, flower arranging, reading, writing and music are more rewarding and conducive to happiness and recovery than passive recreations and spectator sports.

THE BOTTOM LINE

Participation can be healing and enjoyable

Words of reassurance

The music that can deepest reach, and cure all ill,
is cordial speech.

Ralph Waldo Emerson, 1803–82, The Conduct of Life

Words of reassurance

We all talk silently to ourselves on a regular basis in the form of internal dialogue. The words we use play a major role in dictating how we feel. You can raise your self-esteem in these difficult times by using words of reassurance, instead of doubting or criticising yourself.

THE BOTTOM LINE

Speak kindly to yourself

Seize the initiative

Every day, in every way, I'm getting better and better...

Emil Coué, 1857–1926
De la suggestion et de ses applications

Seize the initiative

Whenever you detect an improvement in your condition – no matter how minor or trivial - seize the initiative to fuel your further recovery. Repeat the following words over and over again to yourself emphatically and with conviction: "Every day, in every way, I'm getting better and better."

THE BOTTOM LINE

Fuel your recovery with words

Cause and effect

There's only one corner of the universe you can be certain of improving, and that's your own self.

Aldous Huxley, 1894–1963

Cause and effect

What improvements would you like to see in the quality of your life? What changes would need to take place to make this possible? Develop respect for the universal law of cause and effect - the empowering conviction that we all ultimately direct our own lives - and anything is possible.

THE BOTTOM LINE

We are masters of our own destiny

Have faith in yourself

Great emergencies and crises show us how much greater our vital resources are than we had supposed.

William James, 1842–1910, A letter from William James to W. Lutoslawski dated May 6th, 1906

Have faith in yourself

Serious illness, by its very nature, often subjects us to discomfort, anxiety, and frustration; but you can use this misfortune to your advantage by developing trust in your ability to make the very best recovery available to you.

THE BOTTOM LINE

Believe in *Y-O-U!*

Live in the present day

If we open a quarrel between the past and the present, we shall find that we have lost the future.

Sir Winston Churchill, 1874–1965, From a speech in the House of Commons, June 18th, 1940

Live in the present day

Avoid worrying about what may or may not happen in the future and stop beating yourself up over past mistakes, embarrassments, and regrets. Make today the day you resolve to live in the present day.

THE BOTTOM LINE

Make the best of today

Calm your mind

What I dream of is an art of balance, of purity and serenity... a soothing, calming influence on the mind, rather like a good armchair which provides relaxation from physical fatigue.

Matisse, 1869–1954, Notes d'un peintre

Calm your mind

When you feel tension mounting, pick up a pen and note down what you believe to be the root cause of the problem. Now you have an entry on a piece of paper, rather than a cloud of anxiety hovering over you. Relax, taking three slow, deep breaths and treat yourself to serene and soothing thoughts; focusing your attention on something or someone special.

THE BOTTOM LINE

Relax... Relieve tension

Laughter

Men will confess to treason, murder, arson, false teeth, or a wig. How many of them will own up to a lack of humour?

Frank Colby, 1865–1925, Essays

Laughter

Laughter raises our spirits and brings relief from pain by releasing endorphins, the body's natural painkillers, into the bloodstream. It exercises the lungs and tones the entire cardiovascular system, stimulating blood cells and antibodies. Patients who retain (or develop) their sense of humour in times of stress tend to recover more easily.

THE BOTTOM LINE

Comedy is medicine

Experiencing the moment

Action is consolatory. It is the enemy of thought and the friend of flattering illusions.

Joseph Conrad, 1857–1924, Nostromo

Experiencing the moment

Regretting the past and wishing away the future are devices that people use to evade the reality of the present when misfortune strikes; but there is only one moment in which you can experience life and that is now because anything else is either the past or the future.

THE BOTTOM LINE

Make the best of *NOW*

Take advantage of misfortune

The happiest people seem to be those who have no particular reason for being happy except that they are happy.

Dean W R Inge, 1860–1954,
Wit and Wisdom of Dean Inge, ed. James Marchant

Take advantage of misfortune

One of the few advantages of serious illness is that it forces us to value our health and to take stock of our lives. No matter how unlikely it may seem at this moment, within this calamity could be the key to a happier, more contented future.

THE BOTTOM LINE

Benefit from misfortune

Wisdom in later years

I love everything that's old: old friends, old times, old manners, old books, old wines.

Oliver Goldsmith, 1728–1774, She Stoops to Conquer

Wisdom in later years

You are never too old to recover and the older generation can be a wily lot: they have known tough times before! They have recourse to a lifetime of experience and wisdom and can draw upon this valuable reserve. In the UK, Age Concern is just a telephone call away on 0800 009966 if assistance is needed.

THE BOTTOM LINE

You are never too old to get better

Health is not everything

Each player must accept the cards life deals him or her. But once they are in hand, he or she alone must decide *how to play the cards...*

Voltaire, 1694–1778

Health is not everything

OK, so your health may have taken a pounding, but this doesn't wipe you out as a person. The damage to your health cannot destroy the richness in other areas of your life.

THE BOTTOM LINE

All is not lost: you are still in the game

The colour of life

One should sympathise with the joy, the beauty, the colour of life - the less said about life's sores the better.

Oscar Wilde, 1854–1900, A Woman of no importance

The colour of life

Try focusing your attention, not on what is ailing you, but towards the more colourful and satisfying things in life. Recall your friends and loved ones, your treasured memories, your favourite foods, your dreams and hopes for the future.

THE BOTTOM LINE

Look for the richness in your life

My special place

My special place. It's a place no amount of hurt and anger can deface. I put things back together there; it all falls right in place - in my special space. My special place.

Joni Mitchell, b.1943, song: My special place

My special place

We all need a special place to escape from reality from time to time and you can conjure one up in your imagination if you wish. This inner sanctuary is for you to visualise and visit however and whenever you see fit, perhaps to seek peace, to meditate, or simply to relax.

THE BOTTOM LINE

Experiment with your imagination

Give yourself direction

I felt as if I were walking with destiny, and that my past life had been but a preparation for this hour and this trial... I was sure I should not fail.

Sir Winston Churchill, 1874–1965
The Gathering Storm

Give yourself direction

When you commit yourself to a specific direction in life, your sense of focus, dedication, participation, fulfilment and powers of belief and recovery come alive and life becomes exciting again. What a glorious feeling this is!

THE BOTTOM LINE

You're the boss! Decide your future direction

Find your purpose

This is the true joy in life... being used for a purpose recognised by yourself as a mighty one... being thoroughly worn out before you are thrown on the scrap heap... Being a force of nature instead of a feverish selfish little clod of ailments and grievances complaining that the world will not devote itself to making you happy.

George Bernard Shaw, 1856–1950
Man and Superman

Find your purpose

Nature, in all its functions, is extraordinarily purposeful. Who could possibly imagine that he or she was born into this world for no purpose? Decide on your unique purpose in life and make it happen. Nothing will keep you more alive.

THE BOTTOM LINE

Rediscover, or find a purpose for your life

Perseverance

Perseverance is more prevailing than violence; and many things which cannot be overcome when they are together, yield themselves up when taken little by little.

Plutarch, circa 46–120 AD, Life of Sertorius

Perseverance

Perseverance is a great power and it is freely available to anyone. To benefit, all you have to do is to refuse to give up. On the proviso that what you are actively seeking is attainable - albeit total recovery, the perfect lover, or a new direction in life - press on towards it (making adjustments in your approach, if necessary) and you will be rewarded.

THE BOTTOM LINE

It is always too soon to give up

Siesta

God bless the inventor of sleep, the cloak that covers all men's thoughts, the food that cures all hunger... the balancing weight that levels the shepherd with the king and the simple with the wise.

Miguel Cervantes, 1547–1616, Don Quixote

Siesta

When convalescing, the Mediterranean habit of taking a nap after lunch can be beneficial. During certain cycles of sleep hormones are released into the bloodstream to facilitate essential self-maintenance and repair work throughout our bodies, boosting recovery.

THE BOTTOM LINE

Sleep is nature's gentle nurse at work

Pleasant surprises

Some patients, though conscious that their condition is perilous, recover their health simply through their contentment with the goodness of the physician.

Hippocrates, circa 460–377 BC

Pleasant surprises

What looks grim today because of your particular situation might turn out to be more promising tomorrow. Like the English weather, life has a tendency to come up with the occasional pleasant surprise!

THE BOTTOM LINE

Look on the bright side

Empowering support

A faithful friend is the medicine of life.

Ecclesiasticus 6:16

Empowering support

Cultivate the sort of friends who make you feel good about yourself and who encourage you to reach for the very best recovery available to you. In hospital, if you have nobody to visit you, ask the nurse to arrange for a volunteer visitor. Some people are born to be carers and would welcome the opportunity to make a new friend.

THE BOTTOM LINE

Reach out for support

Enthusiasm

Over the piano was printed a notice: please do not
shoot the pianist. He is doing his best.

Oscar Wilde, 1854–1900, Impression of America
"Leadville"

Enthusiasm

Life is at its richest, and recovery at its most potent, when approached with enthusiasm. If illness or impediment is sapping your day-to-day zest for life, direct your mind to activities that will please you.

THE BOTTOM LINE

Please yourself

Desire

The follies that a man regrets most are those, *which he didn't commit when he had the opportunity.*

Helen Rowland, 1875–1950, A Guide to Men

Desire

Giving yourself a desirable and attainable reason to get well adds new momentum to the need for recovery and is the closest you get to therapy in the fast lane.

THE BOTTOM LINE

Desire is a powerful stimulus

Add variety to life

Do what you can, with what you have,
with where you are now.

Theodore Roosevelt, 1858–1919

Add variety to life

Recovering in hospital and convalescing after illness can be boring. Step outside your usual routine by reading different books and magazines, by talking to different people, by painting different pictures and by viewing your life from a different perspective.

THE BOTTOM LINE

Variety is the spice of life

Reap the benefit

The individual who is able to perceive a glimmer of possibility in a situation that seems, at first glance, full of insurmountable obstacles, is the one who is most likely to reap the greatest benefits.

John Paul Getty, 1892–1976

Reap the benefit

Acknowledge the steps you have taken along the way to combat your illness or misfortune and look for ways to benefit from the situation. This setback can and will strengthen your character if and when you are prepared to search for a positive outcome.

THE BOTTOM LINE

Benefit from your experience

144

Self-fulfilling expectations

Nothing extraordinary, great or beautiful is ever accomplished without thinking about it more often and better than others.

> King Louis XIV of France, 1638–1715
> (known to his subjects as the *Sun King*)

Self-fulfilling expectations

Over time, we are liable to become what we think about most: what we anticipate will happen tends to take place in reality. Self-fulfilling expectations are a prime factor in determining the likelihood of total recovery or the final degree of rehabilitation patients can expect following serious illness.

THE BOTTOM LINE

Expect the best

Happiness

The mind is its own place, and in itself can make
heaven of Hell, a hell of Heaven.

John Milton, 1608–1674, Paradise Lost

Happiness

Before my career as a stress counsellor was cut short by stroke, I became aware that many people, rich and poor, healthy and otherwise, see happiness as an objective to be reached one day. Happiness is not a goal; it is a state of mind: a conscious choice to be exercised on a daily basis, starting now.

THE BOTTOM LINE

Choose to be happy

Working from home

Much of the world's work, it has been said, is done by folk who do not feel quite well.

J. K. Galbraith, b.1908, The Age of Uncertainty

Working from home

Instead of seeing the rug being pulled from under us by serious illness or disablement we can learn to dance on the shifting carpet and adapt to our new circumstances by working from home. Opportunities exist, no matter where in the world you live.

THE BOTTOM LINE

Working from home can be enjoyable

Volunteering your help

Be yourself – the self you always wanted
–compassionate to others and at ease with
yourself: worthy and contented, a special person.

David M Hinds, b.1945

Volunteering your help

The Women's Royal Voluntary Service (WRVS) and The National Association of Hospital and Community Friends (NAHCF) provide valuable and much-needed support for patients. Once you are feeling better, why not volunteer to help them carry on the good work? Either organisation would be delighted to hear from you.

THE BOTTOM LINE

Angels do have fun

The farewell quotation

Some books are to be tasted, others to be
swallowed, and some few to be
chewed and digested.

Francis Bacon, 1561–1626, Essays "Of Studies"

Farewell

This little book is to be tucked into whenever you feel the urge.

All the best for a speedy return to health,

David M Hinds
Polperro, Cornwall.

Enjoyed this book?

David M Hinds is available to speak at functions,
to mastermind group or 1-to-1 mentoring sessions
about making the best of a bad situation, or to
motivate patients to make the very best recovery
available to them.

Contact David via Community Health Publishing:
the UK publishers of this book.

Personalised gift wrap dispatch service

Single copies of this book can be inscribed with a personal message to the recipient from the sender, and dispatched next working day to any hospital, nursing home, or address in the UK. One call to our credit/debit card order line is all that's needed:

Telephone: 01503 273074   Fax: 01503 273148

Trade counter

This title is available in packs of 10 and 100 only.

CHP, Crumplehorn Mill, Polperro, Cornwall PL13 2RJ
e-mail: orderline@chpublishing.fslife.co.uk

Health books by the same author

After Stroke, published by Thorsons @ £9.99 with a foreword by Professor Sir Peter J Morris, FRCS, FRS, Nuffield Professor of Surgery at the University of Oxford, is a complete, step-by-step blueprint for getting better. *"Invaluable not only for people who have had a stroke but also for their carers."* … Sir Peter Morris. *"A warm and motivating read."* … The Stroke Association.

Beat Depression, published by Hodder and Stoughton @ £6.99, has generated many letters and e-mails from readers who were moved from the source of their depression to relief by this supportive and patient-orientated book.